The Ultimate Weight Watchers Cookbook

Delicious Weight Watchers Points Plus Recipes

BY

Gordon Rock

Copyright 2015 Gordon Rock

License Notes

No part of this Book can be reproduced in any form or by any means including print, electronic, scanning or photocopying unless prior permission is granted by the author.

All ideas, suggestions and guidelines mentioned here are written for informative purposes. While the author has taken every possible step to ensure accuracy, all readers are advised to follow information at their own risk. The author cannot be held responsible for personal and/or commercial damages in case of misinterpreting and misunderstanding any part of this Book

About the author

Gordon Rock is the author for hundreds of cookbooks on delicious meals that the 'average Joe' can attempt at home. Including, but definitely not limited to, the Amazon Prime bestseller "Smoking Meat: The Essential Guide to Real Barbecue".

Rock is also known for other well-known titles such as "Making Fresh Pasta", "Hot Sauce", "The Paleo Chocolate Lovers" and "Vegan Tacos", just to name a few.

Rock has been nominated for various awards and has recently been offered a 'Question & Answers' column in Food and Wine Magazine that will give him a greater medium to respond to all the queries readers may have after attempting his recipes. He has also been honored by the

Institution of Culinary Excellence for his outstanding recipes.

Gordon Rock grew up in the outskirts of Los Angeles in California, where he graduated from the Culinary Institute of America with honors. He still resides there along with his wife and three kids. He operates a non - profit organization for aspiring cooks who are unable to finance their culinary education and spends practically all his spare time either in the kitchen or around his desk writing.

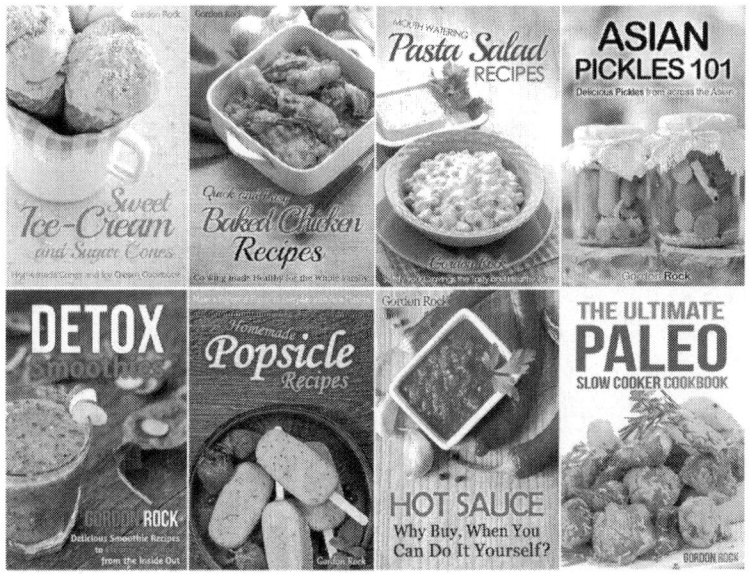

For a complete list of my published books, please, visit my Author's Page...

http://amazon.com/author/gordonrock

Table of Contents

Introduction 7
1. Scrambled Eggs with Scallions and Tomatoes 8
2. Egg and Bacon Burritos 10
3. Chicken Yakitori 13
4. Pumpkin Oatmeal 15
5. Raspberry-Peach Smoothie 17
6. Chicken, tomato and peach couscous salad 19
7. Minted Pea Soup 21
8. Bean and Pepper Salad 23
9. Minted Lentil and Tomato Salad 25
10. Cauliflower Poppers 27
11. Honey Glazed Salmon with Wasabi 29
12. Black Bean Dip 31
13. Grilled Chicken with Key Lime Salsa 33
14. Pumpkin Muffins 35
15. Kale Spinach and Apple Smoothie 37
16. Beetroot Blinis with Garlicky Mushrooms 39
17. Cabbage Soup 41
18. Mexican Chicken 43
19. Baked Spicy French Fries 45
20. Coconut Chicken and Pina colada Dip 47
21. Chocolate Marshmallow Fudge 49
22. Mexican Casserole 51

23. Ginger Berry and oats smoothie 53
24. Spinach Kiwi and Chia Seeds Smoothie 55
25. Chicken Fingers 56
26. Poppy Seed Muffins 58
27. Southwestern Corn 60
28. Quinoa Pilaf 62
29. Cranberry Orange Smoothie 64
30. Garlicky Shrimps 66
Conclusion 68

Introduction

Your weight loss journey requires a lot of dedication and hard work. It is a complete process that is made up of various elements and healthy eating is one of them. It calls for a whole lot of preparation and without it your efforts are likely to go in vain. Healthy eating is not just a menu lined up with healthy food, but it is a lifestyle. You can't lose weight by starving or giving up on your favorite food. But at the same time it is essential that you plan your meals with healthy food items and your intake is in moderation.

This weight watchers cookbook will help you plan your meals. It's a complete guide to a healthy lifestyle, filled with incredibly delicious recipes and less time consuming meals. The right meal combinations contribute significantly in maintaining weight. Not only is your body energized but you are also saved from chronic diseases. This cookbook contains recipes that are made with the essential foods that our body requires to function effectively. You may find some of these recipes mentioned in other publications as the weight watchers magazine also.

You no longer have to put dietary restrictions upon yourself. You simply need to follow the commonly available weight watchers point guide. Each and every recipe in this cookbook will make you satisfied at the end of your last bite. The recipes set out in this book can be followed once you have reached your goal weight. While your weight loss regimen you will not be deprived from the food you love the most. The whole idea of this cookbook is to provide you with a meal plan that you can easily implement in your life and follow till the end.

1. Scrambled Eggs with Scallions and Tomatoes

Eggs are high in protein and a great food for those maintaining their weight. This delicious recipe is perfect for both breakfast and lunch. Recently, the myth stating eggs are bad for your heart has been disproven by scientists, so you can enjoy eggs as much as you want without any guilt.

Servings: ¾ cup per serving

Preparation time: 5 minutes

Points plus value: 3

Calories: 131.9

Fat: 5.6g

Protein: 15.6g

Carbs: 6g

Fiber: 1.2g

Ingredients:

- Eggs, 4
- Egg whites, 4
- Salt, ½ teaspoon
- Fresh tomatoes diced, ¾ cup
- Sliced scallion, 1/3 cup
- Low fat cream cheese, 2 Oz
- Ground black pepper, 1/8 teaspoon
- Cooking spray

Method:

Sprinkle cooking oil over a non-stick pan and coat it. Put over medium heat.

Add all ingredients in a bowl except for cheese and tomatoes. Whisk the mixture until all ingredients are well combined.

Pour the mixture in the pan. When the mixture starts setting turn it with a spatula.

Cut cheese into tiny bits.

Add cheese and tomatoes in the eggs and stir. Keep stirring until the mixture sets. Cook for 1 minute or until a creamy texture is created.

2. Egg and Bacon Burritos

Delicious and healthy tortillas stuffed with bacon and egg,; it's a perfect meal to kick start the day. As long as you have it in moderation, not only is this recipe filling, but gives you plenty of energy to push through the day until lunch.

Servings: 2

Preparation time: 15 minutes

Points plus value: 8

Calories: 500

Fat: 27 g

Protein: 27 g

Carbs: 36 g

Fiber: 1 g

Ingredients:

- Eggs, 2
- Egg whites, 3
- Salt, 1/8 teaspoon
- Finely chopped bacon, 2 slices
- Oregano, ¼ teaspoon
- Black pepper, 1/8 teaspoon
- Low fat sour cream, 4 tablespoon
- Fat-free salsa, 3 tablespoon
- Large wheat flour tortillas, 2
- Ripped medium avocado, 1/8 sliced into wedges
- Cooking spray, butter flavor

Method:

Whisk egg and egg whites together until the mixture becomes foamy.

Add salt, salsa, black pepper, oregano and bacon. Combine all the ingredients well.

Spray the butter flavor cooking spray over a skillet and heat over low flame. Now pour the egg mixture in the skillet and stir while the eggs set. Use a spatula to scramble the eggs.

Preheat oven to 400F.

Spray the cooking spray over a baking tray.

Place half scrambled egg in the center of both tortilla and roll. Don't forget to fold the edges. Now place each tortilla on the baking tray and for 5 minutes.

Top some sour cream and serve with avocado.

3. Chicken Yakitori

This extremely juicy chicken with balanced spices can be served in dinner with lots of salad on side. Known for its distinct flavor, this chicken is a lean meal that is a true delight for your taste buds.

Servings: 4

Preparation time: 15 minutes

Points plus value: 7

Calories: 307.6

Fat: 5.5 g

Protein: 26.6 g

Carbs: 37.1 g

Fiber: 3.8 g

Ingredients:

- Boneless and skinless chicken thighs, all visible fat sheared. 1 lb.
- Mirin, 2 tablespoon
- Garlic clove, 1
- Red bell peppers, diced, 2
- Ginger, minced, 1 teaspoon
- Soy sauce, low sodium, ¼ cup
- Scallions, diced, 8
- Sugar, 2 tablespoon
- Cooked rice, 2 cups

Method:

Cut chicken in 2 inch pieces.

In a medium saucepan mix soy sauce, garlic, sugar, mirin and ginger together and bring to boil. Cook on medium flame for 5 minutes or until the sauce reaches a thick consistency. Now set aside.

Use either a broiler or grill pan. Coat well with cooking spray.

Assemble bell peppers, chicken and scallions on skewer.

Place skewers on the grill pan and brush sauce over chicken repeatedly. Grill until the vegetables become tender and chicken is properly cooked.

Serve warm with rice.

4. Pumpkin Oatmeal

Oats are full of nutritional value. They are perfect to have for breakfast as well as dinner. Not only are they easy to make but with a little creativity you can make different kinds of oatmeal. Also keep in mind that oatmeal is very good for your digestive system.

Servings: 8

Preparation time: 15 minutes

Points plus value: 5

Calories: 277.3

Fat: 4.1 g

Protein: 8.6 g

Carbs: 56.7 g

Fiber: 9 g

Ingredients:

- Oats, steel cut, 1 ½ cup
- Water, 6 cups
- Ground cinnamon, 1 teaspoon
- Uncooked pumpkin, 3 cups
- Nutmeg, grated, ¼ teaspoon
- Honey ½ cup
- Salt, ½ teaspoon

Method:

Steel cut oats take long to cook. It's best if you use a slow cooker.

Put all the ingredients in the cooker and mix well.

Cover the lid and let it cook for 8 hours.

Make sure you mix all the ingredients well before serving.

5. Raspberry-Peach Smoothie

Fruits are not only healthy but they are also your best bet when it comes to satisfy your sweet tooth. Blending these fresh raspberries and peaches with yogurt will make a perfect snack for mid-day hunger.

Servings: 1

Preparation time: 10 minutes

Points plus value: 5

Calories: 190.4

Fat: 1.0 g

Protein: 11.8 g

Carbs: 35.3 g

Fiber: 6.2 g

Ingredients:

- Fat free yogurt, plain, 6oz
- Vanilla extract, ¼ teaspoon
- Raspberries, ½ cup
- No calorie sweetener, ½ teaspoon
- Peach, diced, ½ cup
- Ice cubes, ¼ cup

Method:

In a blender, blend all the ingredients until it reaches a smooth consistency.

Pour in a glass and serve.

6. Chicken, tomato and peach couscous salad

If you are looking for portion control, this recipe will be a great try. The salad contains 300 calories which is a perfect deal for lunch. Tomatoes are high in vitamin D and adding peach to the salad will give a hint of a fruity touch.

Servings: 2

Preparation time: 15 minutes

Points plus value: 4

Calories: 133

Fat: 5 g

Protein: 5 g

Carbs: 26 g

Fiber: 4.5 g

Ingredients:

- Chicken stock, 2/3 cups
- Coriander, chopped, 2 tablespoons
- Spring onion, chopped, 4
- Peach, chopped, 1
- Ground black pepper
- Salt
- Dried couscous, 5 tablespoon
- Cherry tomatoes, halved, 8
- Yellow pepper, diced, ½
- Juice and zest of ½ lemons
- Sliced boneless chicken, ¼ cups

Method:

Take a large bowl and add hot chicken stock, lemon zest, couscous, lemon juice and 1 tablespoon coriander. Cover the bowl with plastic and keep aside for 5 minutes.

Separate the couscous from the mixture in a dish and set aside.

Once the couscous has cooled completely, mix tomatoes, onions, pepper and peaches. Now add chicken pieces and sprinkle the remaining coriander atop.

7. Minted Pea Soup

Tired from the traditional unexciting tomato soup? Try this unique chilled minted pea soup. It's a combination of herbs and vegetables twirling with cream. It can be consumed as an appetizer or a main dish. Any leftover can be refrigerated and can be used later.

Servings: 10

Preparation time: 25 minutes

Points plus value: 3

Calories: 238

Fat: 2 g

Protein: 19 g

Carbs: 38 g

Fiber: 14 g

Ingredients:

- Butter, 2 ½ tablespoon
- Peas, 2 cups
- Chopped shallots, 4
- Pea shoots and double cream
- Mint, chopped, 2-3 tablespoon
- Vegetable stock, 750 ml
- Pinch of sugar

Method:

In a large pan, melt butter over medium flame and add shallots. Cook till they become soft.

Now add stock and peas and boil the soup. Later simmer for 15 minutes to make peas soft. Set aside to cool down.

Pour the soup in a blender along with mint and blend to form puree. Add salt, pepper and sugar according to taste.

Refrigerate until the soup is chilled. Swirl cream and sprinkle pea shoots atop while serving.

8. Bean and Pepper Salad

This is a heavenly protein filled bowl of salad. Loaded with crunchiness of beans and crispiness of pepper it can be consumed as a side salad or main dish. The only time it takes is to cook the peppers, once it's done all you have to do is mix all the ingredients together and you are good to go.

Servings: 8

Preparation time: 1 hour

Points plus value: 6

Calories: 168

Fat: 3.5 g

Protein: 9 g

Carbs: 28.5 g

Fiber: 8 g

Ingredients:

- Red pepper, halved, 2
- Green beans, 2-3 cups
- Yellow peppers, halved, 2
- Salad leaves, 1 cup
- For dressing:
- Olive oil, 6 tablespoon
- Ginger, grated, 1 tablespoon
- Vinegar, 2 tablespoon
- Caster sugar, 1 table spoon

Method:

Preheat the oven to 392C.

Roast the peppers in the oven for 20-25 minutes. Remove the tray when the peppers skin turns slightly char and tightly cover them in a freezer bag to cool. When cooled, peel off the skin and chop the peppers.

Boil the beans in water until they become tender. Drain them under cool water.

Now in a large bowl add all the vegetables and beans.

For dressing, add all the ingredients in the vegetable bowl and toss. Cover the vegetables well in the salad dressing.

9. Minted Lentil and Tomato Salad

This recipe is made up of various mints which add an exciting flavor to it. The secret is to use fresh mint for better flavor and energy. The addition of lentil makes this salad filling and high in protein.

Servings: 6

Preparation time: 15 minutes

Points plus value: 4

Calories: 220

Fat: 9 g

Protein: 10 g

Carbs: 26 g

Fiber: 6 g

Ingredients:

- Dry lentils, 1 cup
- Onions, chopped, ½ cup
- Tomato, diced, 1 cup
- Lemon juice, ¼ cup
- Garlic, minced, 2 teaspoon
- Water, 2 cups
- Celery, chopped, ¼ cup
- Parsley, finely chopped, ½ cup
- Green pepper, chopped, ½ cup
- Salt, ½ teaspoon
- Olive oil, ¼ cup
- Fresh mint, finely chopped, 2 tablespoon

Method:

Boil lentils in water over medium flame. Turn the flame low and cover the pan and cook for 25 minutes. Drain the lentils and set aside in a bowl.

Mix together garlic, parsley, mint, green pepper, onion and celery. Add this to the lentils and toss well.

In a separate bowl, squeeze lemon juice and add salt and olive oil. Mix this with lentils and toss well again. Cover the bowl and refrigerate.

Add tomato before serving.

10. Cauliflower Poppers

Deliciously spicy and crunchy cauliflower can be served with any dip of your choice. It can be included as a side dish or can be eaten as an evening snack. Cauliflower is loaded with health benefits and is a magical vegetable used in weight loss meals.

Servings: 8

Preparation time: 15 minutes

Points plus value: 0

Calories: 19.7

Fat: 0.2 g

Protein: 1.4 g

Carbs: 3.8 g

Fiber: 1.5 g

Ingredients:

- Medium uncooked cauliflower heads, sliced into small bites, 4 cups
- Chili powder, ½ teaspoon
- Salt, ½ teaspoon
- Ground cumin, ½ teaspoon
- Black pepper, ½ teaspoon

Method:

Preheat oven to 400F. Cover the baking tray with cooking spray.

In a medium sized bowl toss cauliflower along with all the spices. Toss until the cauliflowers are well-coated in the spices.

Bake cauliflower for 10 minutes or until they become crunchy.

Serve with a dip of your choice.

11. Honey Glazed Salmon with Wasabi

The tenderizing flavor of salmon prepared with honey and wasabi serves a perfect dinner. It's a filling dish that can be served with cucumber and tomato salad with a little lemon juice mixed to enhance its flavor.

Servings: 4

Preparation time: 25 minutes

Points plus value: 4

Calories: 180.2

Fat: 5.0 g

Protein: 23.7 g

Carbs: 5.9 g

Fiber: 0.2 g

Ingredients:

- Mirin, 3 tablespoons
- Salmon fillet, 4 pieces
- Honey, 1 tablespoon
- Soy sauce, 1 tablespoon
- Scallion, chopped, ¼ cup
- Minced ginger, 1 teaspoon
- Salt, ½ teaspoon
- Black pepper, ½ teaspoon
- Rice vinegar, 1 tablespoon
- Wasabi paste, 2 teaspoons

Method:

Marinate salmon with salt and pepper.

For sauce, boil soy sauce, mirin, wasabi paste, vinegar, ginger and honey in a pan over medium-high flame, stirring occasionally. Set aside when a thick sauce is formed.

Coat a non-stick skillet with cooking spray and put over high flame. Cook salmon till the skin is browned on each side.

Now pour the sauce over salmon and add garnish with scallion.

12. Black Bean Dip

This delicious dip can be served with cauliflower poppers. Exceptionally easy to prepare within very less time, it can also be served with other meals. If you like your food extra spicy all you have to do is mix jalapeno peppers and you are all set.

Servings: 8

Preparation time: 5 minutes

Points plus value: 1

Calories: 249.5

Fat: 1.1 g

Protein: 16.3 g

Carbs: 45.8 g

Fiber: 16.0 g

Ingredients:

- Black beans, 15 oz.
- Salsa, ½ cup
- Ground cumin, 1 teaspoon
- Fat free yogurt, ½ cup
- Salt, ¼ teaspoon
- Cilantro, 1 ½ cup

Method:

Blend all the ingredients in a blender keeping ½ cup cilantro aside for garnishing. Blend till the required consistency is textured.

Garnish with remaining cilantro.

13. Grilled Chicken with Key Lime Salsa

This is another sweet and sour flavored chicken recipe that is perfect for dinner. Chicken takes little time to cook so anyone with an up tight schedule will find this recipe very useful.

Servings: 4

Preparation time: 30 minutes

Points plus value: 5

Calories: 258.8

Fat: 10.6 g

Protein: 24.7 g

Carbs: 16.7 g

Fiber: 2.5 g

Ingredients:

- Chicken breast, 4 pieces
- Oranges, pithed and seeded, 3
- Key lime juice, 3 tablespoons
- Worcestershire sauce, ¼ cup
- Key lime juice, 2 tablespoons
- Green chili, chopped, 1 teaspoon
- Scallions, chopped, 2 tablespoons
- Cilantro, chopped, 1 tablespoon

Method:

Marinate chicken with 3 tablespoon lime juice and Worcestershire sauce and cover tightly in a plastic bag. Refrigerate for 4 hours.

For salsa, mix remaining ingredients well and place in freezer for an hour.

Preheat either a boiler or grill. Cook chicken thoroughly.

Serve with salsa.

14. Pumpkin Muffins

Craving for something sweet? This is an incredible muffin recipe that is prepared with only 3 ingredients and is loaded with awesomeness and deliciousness. It is easy to prepare and can be enjoyed as an evening delight.

Servings: 24

Preparation time: 30 minutes

Points plus value: 2

Calories: 97.6

Fat: 2.9 g

Protein: 1.1 g

Carbs: 17.0 g

Fiber: 0.4 g

Ingredients:

- Cake mix, 1 box
- Pumpkin, 15 oz.
- Water, 1 cup

Method:

Preheat oven for 350F.

Mix the cake mix in water. Pour the mixture in a greased muffin tray.

Bake the muffins for 20-25 minutes or until the toothpick comes out clean.

15. Kale Spinach and Apple Smoothie

Kale and spinach are best known for aiding digestion and cleaning the body. When mixed together with other vegetables and fruits they create a refreshing blend of a healthy smoothie. It's so filling that you won't need a proper meal after it for several hours.

Servings: 1

Preparation time: 5 minutes

Points plus value: 6

Calories: 240

Ingredients:

- Spinach leaves, 1 cup
- Kale leaves, 1 cup chopped
- Frozen banana, 1
- Lite vanilla soy milk, 1 cup
- Apple, ½
- Honey, ½ teaspoon

Method:

Blend kale, vanilla milk and spinach together until no chunks remain.

Now add banana, honey and apple and blend again.

Serve chilled.

16. Beetroot Blinis with Garlicky Mushrooms

Beetroot is loaded with health benefits. It helps greatly in cleansing the blood. Garlic on the other hand also has several healthy properties. When these two ingredients are combined, topped with mushrooms, they form an irresistible meaty meal.

Servings: 30

Preparation time: 30 minutes

Points plus value: 3

Calories: 57

Fat: 3.5 g

Ingredients:

- Buckwheat flour, 1 cup
- Milk, 1 cup
- Butter, 1/2 cup
- Eggs, 2
- Yeast sachet, 1
- For the topping:
- Beetroot, 1 cup
- Ricotta, 125 g
- Butter, 1 ½ cup
- Garlic, finely chopped, 3
- Crème fraiche, 3 tablespoon

- Small bunch of dill, chopped
- Button mushroom, sliced, 1 ½ cup

Method:

In a large bowl mix all ingredients together and leave for 30 minutes.

Melt butter in a saucepan and coat a skillet with it properly.

Add teaspoonful of blini batter into the skillet and cook each side until it changes color.

Blend beetroot, ricotta and crème fraiche in a blender. Don't blend too much forming powder.

Season it and add dill. Set aside to cool down.

In another saucepan, melt butter and fry garlic and mushrooms until they turn golden.

For serving, put cooked blini in a platter top it with beetroot mix and add mushrooms.

Sprinkle the remaining dill for garnish.

Repeat the serving steps with other blini as well.

17. Cabbage Soup

Who doesn't enjoy a bowl of hot soup? Soups are perfect for appetizers and can also be consumed as a proper meal. Cabbage is high in sulfur and has detoxifying properties. This cabbage soup is a delightful healthy treat.

Servings: 6-8

Preparation time: 35 minutes

Points plus value: 0

Calories: 21.9

Fat: 0.1 g

Protein: 0.9 g

Carbs: 4.9 g

Fiber: 1.5 g

Ingredients:

- Nonfat beef broth, 3 cups
- Cabbage, chopped, 2 cups
- Green beans, ½ cup
- Basil, ½ teaspoon
- Tomato paste, 1 tablespoon
- Carrot, chopped, ½ cup
- Garlic cloves, minced, 2
- Yellow onion, ½
- Oregano, ½ teaspoon
- Zucchini, chopped, ½ cup
- Salt and pepper

Method:

Coat a large pot with cooking spray and sauté garlic, onions and carrots for 5 minutes.

Now add broth, cabbage, beans, basil, tomato paste, oregano. Salt and pepper to the sautéed vegetables. Simmer until the vegetables are tender.

Add zucchini and cook for 10 minutes.

Serve hot.

18. Mexican Chicken

Mexican chicken is a hearty dish that is extremely easy to prepare. All you need for this recipe is a handful of ingredients and you are good to go. Sizzling chicken with spicy flavors makes a great dinner meal.

Servings: 4

Preparation time: 35 minutes

Points plus value: 8

Calories: 177.9

Fat: 3.2 g

Protein: 25.8 g

Carbs: 11.4 g

Fiber: 2.7 g

Ingredients:

- Taco seasoning, 1 ¼ oz.
- Salsa, 1 cup
- Fat free sour cream, ¼ cup
- Boneless chicken breast, 4

Method:

Marinate chicken with taco seasoning and keep it in a sealed plastic bag.

Coat a baking dish with cooking spray and place chicken.

Bake at 375 F for 30 minutes. Top the chicken with salsa 5 minutes before taking it out of the oven.

Serve with sour cream on top.

19. Baked Spicy French Fries

French fries are popular among every age group. They have this amazingly delicious taste that pleases everyone. Potatoes are rich in carbohydrates and if baked they can serve with good nutritional value.

Servings: 4

Preparation time: 35 minutes

Points plus value: 3

Calories: 153.4

Fat: 0.3 g

Protein: 5.6 g

Carbs: 32.7 g

Fiber: 4.2 g

Ingredients:

- Egg whites, 2
- Potatoes, 2
- Ground cumin, ¾ teaspoon
- Salt, ½ teaspoon
- Chili powder, ½ teaspoon
- Black pepper, ¼ teaspoon

Method:

Preheat oven to 425 F.

In a bowl mix all ingredients together and toss well.

Coat a baking sheet with cooking spray and place the potatoes in it. Bake till the potatoes turn light golden brown for about 15 minutes.

20. Coconut Chicken and Pina colada Dip

This recipe combines chicken so well with coconut flavor. The dip on the side is another yummy treat. Very easy to cook and filling at the same time, this dish is perfect to serve at dinner.

Servings: 4

Preparation time: 35 minutes

Points plus value: 7

Calories: 296.8

Fat: 6.9 g

Protein: 30.3 g

Carbs: 27.1 g

Fiber: 1.6 g

Ingredients:

- Boneless chicken breast, 4
- Lime juice (fresh), 1 tablespoon
- Light coconut milk, 1 can
- Hot pepper sauce, 1 tablespoon
- Ground black pepper, ¼ teaspoon
- Sweetened flaked coconut, ½ cup
- Breadcrumbs, ¾ cup
- Salt, ½ teaspoon
- For dip:
- Sour cream (Fat free), 3 oz.
- Crushed pineapple, 3oz.
- Nonalcoholic pina colada drink mix, 4 oz.

Method:

Preheat oven at 400F.

Marinate chicken with lime juice, pepper sauce and coconut milk. Pack it in a sealed plastic bag and refrigerate for 1 ½ hours.

In a bowl mix breadcrumbs, salt, pepper and coconut and fold chicken in the mixture properly.

Now coat a baking tray with cooking spray and place chicken in it. Spray some cooking spray on chicken as well and bake for about 30 minutes.

21. Chocolate Marshmallow Fudge

This recipe makes soft and moist fudge that you will love eating. Extremely easy to make and very delicious in taste, it is a perfect delight to serve your chocolate cravings. This recipe is a must try.

Servings: 36

Preparation time: 15-20 minutes

Points plus value: 3

Calories: 100.1

Fat: 5.4 g

Protein: 1.6 g

Carbs: 14.9 g

Fiber: 1.6 g

Ingredients:

- Semisweet chocolate chips, chopped, 1 ½ cups
- Large marshmallows, 14
- Fat free evaporated milk, 2/3 cup
- Sugar, 1 2/3 cups
- Reduced calorie margarine, 2 tablespoons

Method:

In a saucepan mix margarine, sugar and milk. Boil the liquid and cook on low flame for 3 minutes. Keep stirring.

Now add marshmallows and chocolate in the liquid and stir. Remove from flame and keep stirring until it forms a smooth mixture.

Coat a baking pan with cooking spray. Preferably an 8x8 pan. Now pour the chocolate mixture into the pan and even it out. Refrigerate for 2 hours.

Cut into squares and serve.

22. Mexican Casserole

This is a treat for beef lovers. If you are bored of eating chicken every day, try out this simple recipe. It is made up of healthy vegetables and is very filling. The good thing about this recipe is that you can add vegetables of your choice to it.

Servings: 6

Preparation time: 1 hour

Points plus value: 6.5

Calories: 355.4

Fat: 5.8 g

Protein: 26.7 g

Carbs: 52.2 g

Fiber: 10.3 g

Ingredients:

- Extra lean ground beef, 1 lb
- Jalapeno slices chopped, ¼ cup
- Corn, 1 can
- Chopped onion, ½ cup
- Tomatoes chopped, 2 cups
- Corn tortillas, 8
- Black beans, 1 can

- Nonfat sour cream, ¾ cup
- Taco seasoning mix, 1 package
- Cilantro chopped, 1/3 bunch
- Reduced-fat Mexican cheese blend, shredded, 1/3 cup

Method:

Cook beef with onions in a skillet. When the beef turns brown completely add corn, tomatoes, jalapenos, taco seasoning and beans. Mix the ingredients well and cook for 5 minutes.

Coat a baking dish with nonstick cooking spray and cut tortillas in half and place on the dish.

Put teaspoonful of beef mixture over the tortillas. Now spread cream over it. Put remaining tortillas and mixture as a second coat and cover the dish with plastic and refrigerate.

Preheat oven to 350F.

Bake beef mixture for 25 minutes. Add cheese and bake for another 5 minutes to melt the cheese.

Serve with cilantro, olives, and tomatoes.

23. Ginger Berry and oats smoothie

This is a low calorie diet smoothie. Oats are widely used to reduce weight and have multiple benefits. The sweetness of berries will neutralize the strong flavors of ginger. From its color to its taste, this recipe is a hit.

Servings: 1-2

Preparation time: 10 minutes

Calories: 179

Points plus value: 4

Ingredients:

- Prepared oatmeal, ¼ cup
- Ginger, grated, ½ teaspoon
- Low-fat milk, ¼ cup
- Honey, 1 teaspoon
- Strawberries, ½ cup
- Ice, ½ cup
- Fresh blackberries, ½ cup

Method:

Cut strawberries into small pieces.

Add all the ingredients in a blender and blend well until the desired consistency is achieved without and lumps

Serve immediately.

24. Spinach Kiwi and Chia Seeds Smoothie

Chia seeds are another magical ingredient that aids in weight loss. This is a healthy green smoothie with low calories and makes a great snack. Kiwi adds that exceptional tartness to it with bananas making it moderately sweet and thick.

Servings: 1-2

Preparation time: 10 minutes

Points plus value: 6

Calories: 226

Ingredients:

- Almond milk, 1 ½ cups
- Banana, 1
- Baby spinach leaves, 1 ½ cups
- Ripe kiwi, 1
- Chia seeds, 2 tablespoons

Method:

Cut banana and kiwi into small chunks. Make sure u use a frozen banana.

Blend all the ingredients in a blender until smooth.

Add ice and blend again. Serve immediately.

25. Chicken Fingers

Crispy and crunchy chicken fingers make a delicious side dish. Very easy to prepare in very less time, they can also be consumed as snacks during midday. Enjoy it with a honey mustard dip to enhance the taste.

Servings: 4

Preparation time: 15 minutes

Points plus value: 6

Calories: 265.1

Fat: 12.1 g

Protein: 20.0 g

Carbs: 18.2 g

Fiber: 0.5 g

Ingredients:

- Chicken strips, 4
- Crushed corn flakes, ½ cup
- Honey, 2 tablespoon
- Beaten egg whites, 2
- Dijon mustard, 2 tablespoon
- Basil, 1 teaspoon

Method:

Preheat oven at 400F.

Mix basil and corn flakes in a bowl.

Coat chicken strips in beaten egg whites and fold in crushed corn flakes. Repeat this with other chicken strips.

Coat a baking sheet with cooking spray and place chicken strips into it.

Bake for 12 minutes.

Mix mustard and honey for dip sauce.

26. Poppy Seed Muffins

This is another delightful muffin recipe made with poppy seeds. This is prepared in very little time with very few ingredients that are easily available in your pantry. Poppy seeds are also great for weight loss and are used widely in different dishes.

Servings: 12

Preparation time: 25 minutes

Points plus value: 2 per muffin

Calories: 197.8

Fat: 8.1 g

Protein: 3.7 g

Carbs: 27.5 g

Fiber: 0.8 g

Ingredients:

- Poppy seeds, 1 tablespoon
- Flour, 1 ¾ cup
- Baking powder, 2 ½ teaspoons
- Butter, 2 tablespoons
- Lemon zest, 1 tablespoons
- Baking soda, ½ teaspoon
- Egg, 1
- Low-fat buttermilk, 1 ¼ cups
- Sugar, ¾ cup
- Salt, ½ teaspoon

Method:

Preheat oven at 400F.

Mix flour and all the ingredients in a bowl. Make a well in the center of the mixture and pour egg, butter and buttermilk.

Combine it all together and make a thick batter.

Grease muffin tray and put tablespoonful into each cup.

Bake for 20 minutes.

27. Southwestern Corn

Corn is another favorite of everyone. Prepared within minutes, this dish can be served as a sideline with almost every meal. It can also be eaten as a snack. Corn is a low calorie snack so you can enjoy it as much as you want.

Servings: 4

Preparation time: 18 minutes

Points plus value: 4

Calories: 195.3

Fat: 5.0 g

Protein: 4.6 g

Carbs: 36.7 g

Fiber: 5.5 g

Ingredients:

- Frozen corn, 1 can
- Medium poblano chilies, 2
- Red onion, chopped, 1
- Vegetable oil, 1 tablespoon
- Cumin, ½ teaspoon
- Hominy, 1 can
- Lime, 1
- Salt
- Cilantro, chopped, 3 tablespoons
- Lime juice, 1 ½ tablespoons
- Oregano, ½ teaspoon
- Garlic cloves, chopped, 2

Method:

Broil chilies directly over flame until the skin turns char. Put them aside in a plastic bag to cool down. After 10 minutes deseed the chilies and roughly chop them.

Sauté onions in vegetable oil over medium flame. Add garlic, oregano and cumin and cook for further 2 minutes.

Now mix hominy and corn while stirring time to time. Now add chopped chilies and salt and cook for another 3 minutes.

Put the prepared corn in a bowl and garnish with cilantro and lime juice.

28. Quinoa Pilaf

It is sweet and tender pea quinoa that is deliciously spiced with lemon and pepper. It is perfect for those who love rice as it is a great substitute for rice. It truly makes a delicious lunch meal.

Servings: 3

Preparation time: 30 minutes

Points plus value: 5

Calories: 134.6

Fat: 3.3 g

Protein: 5.0 g

Carbs: 21.5 g

Fiber: 2.9 g

Ingredients:

- Quinoa, ½ cup
- Peas, ½ cup
- Onion, chopped, ½
- Carrots, finely chopped, 2
- Celery stalk, 1
- Bay leaf, 1
- Lemon rind grated, 1
- Lemon juice, 1 tablespoon
- Butternut squash, diced, 1 cup
- Vegetable stock, 1 cup
- Salt and pepper, to taste
- Olive oil, 1 tablespoon

Method:

Cook celery, carrots and onion in oil over medium flame.

Rinse and drain quinoa and add to the vegetables. Cook for 2 minutes

Now add squash, bay leaf, lemon juice and rind along with some water and boil.

Now cover the pan and simmer for 20 minutes or until quinoa becomes tender.

Remove bay leafs and add peas. Add salt and pepper.

29. Cranberry Orange Smoothie

This recipe is a combination of cranberries, orange and banana that is rich in vitamin C and fiber. Not only does it provide energy but it is also extremely refreshing with a great hint of sweetness and tartness.

Servings: 2

Preparation time: 5 minutes

Points plus value: 5

Calories: 129

Ingredients:

- Cranberry juice, ¾ cup
- Frozen banana, ½
- Orange, 1
- Cinnamon, 1/8 teaspoon
- Nonfat yogurt, ¾ cup
- Frozen berries, ¾ cup
- Vanilla extract, 1/8 teaspoon

Method:

Peel orange and slice into small chunks.

Cut banana into small pieces.

Add all the ingredients in a blender and blend until no chunks remain.

Add ice and blend again,

Serve immediately.

30. Garlicky Shrimps

This recipe is a blend of sweet and spicy flavors. These shrimps are easy to make and incredible in taste. Serve this recipe with noodles on the side. It is a perfect treat to be enjoyed at dinner.

Servings: 4

Preparation time: 30 minutes

Points plus value: 5

Calories: 200.2

Fat: 6.7 g

Protein: 21.4 g

Carbs: 12.5 g

Fiber: 0.8 g

Ingredients:

- Shrimps, deveined and peeled, 1 ¼ lbs.
- Lemon rind, grated, 1 teaspoon
- Olive oil, 4 teaspoon
- Breadcrumbs, ½ cup
- Garlic cloves, minced, 3
- Lemon juice, 2 tablespoon
- Salt, ¼ teaspoon
- Chopped parsley, 3 tablespoon

Method:

Preheat oven at 400F.

Take 4 gratin dishes and grease with cooking spray.

In a bowl mix breadcrumbs, oil and remaining ingredients together.

Fold shrimps in the breadcrumbs mixture and place into the baking dish.

Bake for 15 minutes or till shrimps turn light brown.

Conclusion

Planning your meals is the most crucial part of any weight loss regimen. Coming up with different ideas almost every day is next to impossible. According to a survey, people quit their weight loss journey in between for the very same reason that they get bored eating the same kind of meals every day. Their busy schedule does not allow them to spend lots of time preparing food.

Healthy eating not only contributes in weight loss but it also helps your body function effectively. Healthy eating is more like a lifestyle, a lifestyle that promotes positive wellbeing. It is very necessary that we add certain vegetables and fruits in our daily intake. But then again the question arises, 'what are those particular vegetables and fruits?'

To make your life easier, we have combined several recipes in one place and provided them to you in this weight watchers cookbook. Each one of these recipes is loaded with several health benefits that you may find in some weight watchers magazines.

Every single ingredient that helps promote health is mentioned in this cookbook and you can mark it accordingly in your weight watchers point guide. You no longer have to follow a mundane eating routine. This weight watchers cookbook contains everything in it, from breakfast ideas to lunch, dinner, salad and snacks; you will find it all.

Now free yourself from excuses and try out these simple and easy recipes. Remember! You can only achieve what you work hard for, and in order to get in shape you need to work hard and follow a proper eating routine.

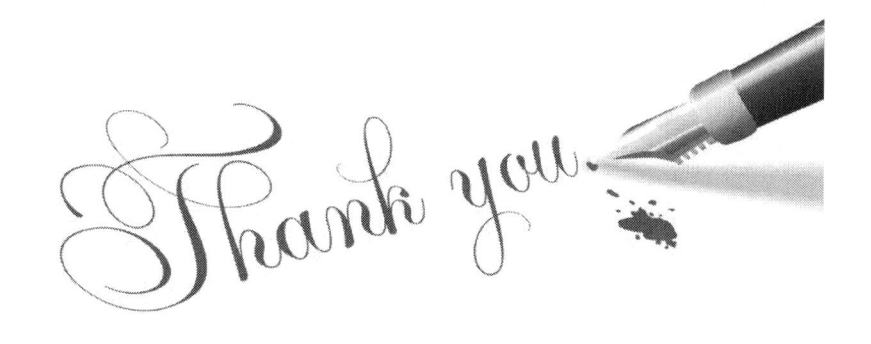

Thank you for reading my book. Your feedback is important to me. It would be greatly appreciated if you could please take a moment to REVIEW this book on Amazon so that we could make our next version better

Thanks!

Gordon Rock
bunsomsaetow@gmail.com

Made in the USA
Lexington, KY
01 November 2015